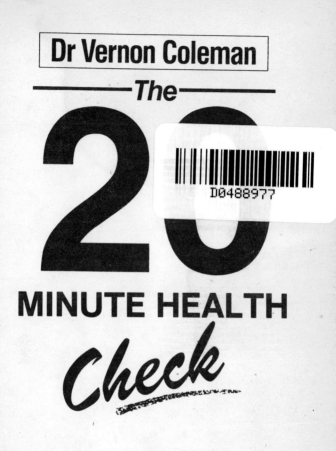

# Dr Vernon Coleman

## The

# 20

## MINUTE HEALTH

## Check

A STAR BOOK
*published by*
the Paperback Division of
W H Allen & Co Plc

A Star Book
Published in 1989
by the Paperback Division of
W. H. Allen & Co Plc
44 Hill Street, London W1X 8LB

Copyright © Dr Vernon Coleman 1989
Design Cecil Smith

Typeset by Avocet Marketing Services, Bicester, Oxon
Printed and bound in Great Britain by
Cox & Wyman Ltd, Reading

ISBN 0 352 32304 3

Dedicated to the memory of my
grandparents.

# CONTENTS

## PART 1

## PART 2

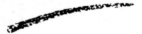

## PART I

# The
# 20
# MINUTE HEALTH
# Check

# INTRODUCTION

*The 20 minute health check* is a comprehensive screening programme designed to test every aspect of your lifestyle – from your eating habits to your susceptibility to stress.

As you work your way through the 120 questions listed here you will collect points that will not only give you an automatic health check – they will also tell you if your lifestyle is likely to lead to any particular health problems.

The seven specific disorders included are:

- Heart disease and circulatory problems (H)
- Respiratory disease (R)
- Digestive problems (D)
- Cancer (C)
- Muscle and joint problems (J)
- Stress susceptibility (S)
- Alcohol consumption (A)

When you have completed the questions add up your totals and turn to p. 26 to find out exactly what your score means.

**1** Do you deliberately exercise every day, or nearly every day (at least five days per week)?
Yes: Score 4 and go to 3
No: Score 1 and go to 2

**2** Do you ever deliberately exercise?
Yes: Score 2 and go to 3
No: Score 1 and go to 18

**3** When you take exercise, do you usually try to push yourself through the pain barrier?
Yes: Score 1, H3 and J5 and go to 4
No: Score 4 and go to 4

**4** Do you enjoy your exercise?
Yes: Score 2 and go to 5
No: Score 1 and H2 and go to 5

**5** If you get a pain, do you always stop your exercise?
Yes: Score 5 and go to 6
No: Score 1, H3 and J5 and go to 6

**6** Have you ever suffered from any injury or illness caused by exercise?
Yes: Score 1 and J3 and go to 7
No: Score 2 and go to 7

**7** Do you ever introduce a sense of competitiveness into your exercise (e.g. running against the clock or playing sports where there are winners and losers)?
Yes: Go to 8
No: Score 1 and go to 9

**8** Do you ever worry about failing or losing?
Yes: Score H1 and go to 9
No: Score 1 and go to 9

**9** Are you receiving medical attention for any problem?
Yes: Go to 10
No: Score 4 and go to 12

**10** Have you consulted your doctor about your exercise programme?
Yes: Score 2 and go to 11
No: Score 2 and go to 12

**11** Has he given you permission to continue exercising?
Yes: Score 2 and go to 12
No: Go to 12

**12** Do you usually exercise with other people?
Yes: Go to 13
No: Score 5 and go to 14

**13** Have two or more of them been injured or made ill by exercise in the last 12 months?
Yes: Score 3, H1 and J2 and go to 14
No: Score 6 and go to 14

**14** Do you take care to buy and wear good equipment?
Yes: Score 3 and go to 15
No: Score 1 and J3 and go to 15

**15** Do you ever jog or run on hard pavements or roads?
Yes: Score 1 and J4 and go to 16
No: Score 6 and go to 25

**16** Does your jogging or running take you along roads on which there is heavy traffic?
Yes: Score 1 and go to 17
No: Score 2 and go to 17

**17** Do you regularly jog or run along cambered roads?
Yes: Score 1 and J3 and go to 25
No: Score 2 and go to 25

**18** Do you regularly suffer from ill health?
Yes: Score 4 and go to 19
No: Score 8 and go to 20

**19** Do you think that your failure to exercise could be responsible for your poor health?
Yes: Score 2 and go to 20
No: Score 4 and go to 20

**20** Do you get breathless if you have to exercise unexpectedly?
Yes: Score 4 and R6 and go to 21
No: Score 6 and go to 21

**21** Do you worry about being out of shape?
Yes: Score 1 and H2 and go to 22
No: Score 2 and go to 22

**22** Do you feel guilty about not exercising?
Yes: Score 1 and go to 23
No: Score 2 and go to 23

**23** Does your lack of exercise affect your ability to enjoy life?
Yes: Score 3 and go to 24
No: Score 5 and go to 24

**24** Has your doctor told you to exercise?
Yes: Score 2 and go to 26
No: Score 4 and go to 26

**25** Were you instructed to exercise by your doctor?
Yes; Score 2 and go to 26
No: Score 3 and go to 26

**26** Are you more than 14 lbs overweight? (see weight tables p. 88 / 90)
Yes: Score 10, H2, R2, D2 and J4 and go to 27
No: Score 40 and go to 29

**27** Are you more than 28 lbs overweight?
Yes: Score H1, R1, D1 and J3 and go to 28
No: Score 20 and go to 30

**28** Are you more than 56 lbs overweight?
Yes: Score H2, R2, D2 and J6 and go to 30
No: Score 10 and go to 30

**29** Are you more than 14 lbs underweight?
Yes: Go to 30
No: Score 10 and go to 30

**30** Does your weight affect your relationships with people you meet?
Yes: Score 5 and go to 31
No: Score 7 and go to 31

**31** Does your weight affect the clothes you wear?
Yes: Score 3 and go to 32
No: Score 5 and go to 32

**32** Does your weight ever embarrass you?
Yes: Go to 33
No: Score 5 and go to 33

**33** Does your weight affect your sex life?
Yes: Go to 34
No: Score 5 and go to 34

**34** Does your weight depress you?
Yes: Score 3 and go to 35
No: Score 6 and go to 35

**35** Do you think your weight is having an effect on your health or do you suffer from any disease related to your weight?
Yes: Score 6, H3, R3, D3 and J7 and go to 36
No: Score 12 and go to 36

**36** Has your doctor ever told you to lose weight?
Yes; Score 5, H2, R2, D2 and J5 and go to 37
No: Score 10 and go to 38

**37** Are you currently following his instructions?
Yes: Score 3 and go to 38
No: Go to 38

**38** Is your father still alive?
Yes: Go to 39
No: Go to 44

**39** Does he suffer from heart disease?
Yes: Score H2 and go to 40
No: Score 2 and go to 40

**40** Does he suffer from diabetes?
Yes: Go to 41
No: Score 2 and go to 41

**41** Does he suffer from high blood pressure?
Yes: Score H1 and go to 42
No: Score 2 and go to 42

**42** Was he born with any serious disorder or
disease?
Yes: Go to 43
No: Score 2 and go to 43

**43** Does he suffer from peptic ulceration?
Yes: Score D3 and go to 49
No: Score 2 and go to 49

**44** Did he suffer from heart disease?
Yes: Score H2 and go to 45
No: Score 2 and go to 45

**45** Did he suffer from diabetes?
Yes: Go to 46
No: Score 2 and go to 46

**46** Did he suffer from high blood pressure?
Yes: Score H1 and go to 47
No: Score 2 and go to 47

**47** Was he born with any serious disorder or disease?
Yes: Go to 48
No: Score 2 and go to 48

**48** Did he suffer from peptic ulceration?
Yes: Score D3 and go to 50
No: Score 2 and go to 50

**49** Choose which of these statements is true:
He is 70 years of age or less: Score 16 and go to 51
He is between 71 and 80 years of age: Score 18 and go to 51
He is 81 years of age or older: Score 20 and go to 51

**50** Choose which of these statements is true:
He died under the age of 50: Score 10 and go to 51
He died between the ages of 50 and 60: Score 12 and go to 51
He died between the ages of 61 and 70: Score 14 and go to 51
He died between the ages of 71 and 80: Score 18 and go to 51
He died at the age of 81 or more: Score 20 and go to 51

**51** Is your mother still alive?
Yes: Go to 52
No: Go to 57

**52** Does she suffer from heart disease?
Yes: Score H2 and go to 53
No: Score 2 and go to 53

**53** Does she suffer from diabetes?
Yes: Go to 54
No: Score 2 and go to 54

**54** Does she suffer from high blood pressure?
Yes: Score H1 and go to 55
No: Score 2 and go to 55

**55** Was she born with any serious disorder or disease?
Yes: Go to 56
No: Score 2 and go to 56

**56** Does she suffer from peptic ulceration?
Yes: Score D3 and go to 62
No: Score 2 and go to 62

**57** Did she suffer from heart disease?
Yes: Score H2 and go to 58
No: Score 2 and go to 58

**58** Did she suffer from diabetes?
Yes: Go to 59
No: Score 2 and go to 59

**59** Did she suffer from high blood pressure?
Yes: Score H1 and go to 60
No: Score 2 and go to 60

**60** Was she born with any serious disorder or disease?
Yes: Go to 61
No: Score 2 and go to 61

**61** Did she suffer from peptic ulceration?
Yes: Score D3 and go to 63
No: Score 2 and go to 63

**62** Choose which of these statements is true:
She is 70 years of age or under: Score 16 and go to 64
She is between 71 and 80 years of age: Score 18 and go to 64
She is 81 years of age or older; Score 20 and go to 64

**63** Choose which of these statements is true:
She died under the age of 50: Score 10 and go to 64
She died between the ages of 50 and 60: Score 12 and go to 64
She died between the ages of 61 and 70: Score 14 and go to 64
She died between the ages of 71 and 80: Score 18 and go to 64
She died at the age of 81 or more: Score 20 and go to 64

**64** Do you suffer from any specific disease and/or symptoms which could be related to your eating habits?
Yes: Go to 65
No: Score 12 and go to 67

**65** Have you needed to ask for professional advice about your eating habits?
Yes: Go to 66
No: Score 4 and go to 67

**66** Do you (or did you) follow the advice you were given?
Yes: Score 8 and go to 67
No: Score 4 and go to 67

**67** Do you suffer from high blood pressure?
Yes: Score 2 and go to 68
No: Score 8 and go to 69

**68** Do you limit your intake of salt?
Yes: Score 4 and go to 69
No: Score 2 and H4 and go to 69

**69** Do you suffer from heart disease and/or any arterial problems?
Yes: Score 4 and H4 and go to 70
No: Score 6 and go to 71

**70** Do you limit your intake of animal fats such as butter & cream?
Yes: score 15 and go to 72
No: Score 5, H12 and D4 and go to 72

**71** Do you limit your intake of animal fats such as butter & cream?
Yes: Score 15 and go to 72
No: Score 7, H10 and D4 and go to 72

**72** Do any particular foods disagree with you?
Yes: Score 3 and D4 and go to 73
No: Score 9 and go to 74

**73** Do you avoid those foods whenever possible?
Yes: Score 4 and go to 74
No: Score D6 and go to 74

**74** Do you suffer from a food allergy?
Yes: Score 2 and go to 75
No: Score 7 and go to 76

**75** Do you avoid the food(s) to which you are allergic?
Yes: Score 4 and go to 76
No: Score 2 and go to 76

**76** Do you eat regular amounts of roughage or bran?
Yes: Score 10 and go to 77
No: Score 7 and D6 and go to 77

**77** Do you eat a normal, well-balanced diet which includes meat, vegetables, fruit and cereals?
Yes: Score 14 and go to 78
No: Score 4 and go to 78

**78** Do you follow a diet which means excluding certain types of food (e.g. are you a vegetarian)?
Yes: Score 4 and go to 79
No: Score 7 and go to 80

**79** Do you take particular care to ensure that your body is not deprived of essential nutrients?
Yes: Score 3 and go to 80
No: Score 1 and go to 80

**80** Have you ever suffered from any disease associated with an inadequate diet (e.g. scurvy, iron deficiency, anaemia etc)?
Yes: Score 3 and go to 81
No: Score 12 and go to 82

**81** Have you changed your eating habits to ensure that this problem does not recur?
Yes: Score 9 and go to 82
No: Go to 82

**82** Do you smoke?
Yes: Go to 83
No: Score 95 and go to 94

**83** Do you smoke a pipe only?
Yes: Score 40 and go to 88
No: Go to 84

**84** Do you smoke between 1 and 20 cigarettes a day (or cigar equivalent)?
Yes: Score 25, C6, H1, R8 and D1 and go to 86
No: Go to 85

**85** Do you smoke less than 40 cigarettes a day (or cigar equivalent)?
Yes: Score 20, C12, H2, R16 and D2 and go to 86
No: Score 16, C16, H4, R24 and D4 and go to 86

**86** Do you smoke tipped cigarettes?
Yes: Score 5 and go to 87
No: Score C5, H1, R2 and D1 and go to 87

**87** Do you have nicotine stained fingers and/or do you smoke down to the butt?
Yes: Score C5, H1, R2, D1 and go to 88
No: Score 5 and go to 88

**88** Do you have a regular and/or persistent cough?
Yes: Score C4 and R4 and go to 89
No: Score 5 and go to 89

**89** Do you suffer from breathlessness?
Yes: Score R4 and go to 90
No: Score 5 and go to 90

**90** Do you suffer from frequent chest infections or bronchitis?
Yes: Score R4 and go to 91
No: Score 5 and go to 91

**91** Do you suffer from heart disease or high blood pressure?
Yes: Score H4 and go to 92
No: Score 5 and go to 92

**92** Do you suffer from any stomach disorder?
Yes: Score D4 and go to 93
No: Score 5 and go to 93

**93** Has a doctor advised you to give up smoking?
Yes: Go to 94
No: Score 5 and go to 94

**94** Do you drink alcohol for comfort?
Yes: Score A1, C1 and D1 and go to 95
No: Score 5 and go to 95

**95** Do you drink secretly?
Yes: Score A1, C1 and D1 and go to 96
No: Score 5 and go to 96

**96** Do you feel guilty about your drinking?
Yes: Score A1, C1 and D1 and go to 97
No: Score 5 and go to 97

**97** Has the quality of your work gone down because of your drinking?
Yes: Score A1, C1 and D1 and go to 98
No: Score 5 and go to 98

**98** Is your capacity to work worse after lunch because of drinking?
Yes: Score A1, C1 and D1 and go to 99
No: Score 5 and go to 99

**99** Do you find yourself having to make excuses because of your drinking?
Yes: Score A1, C1 and D1 and go to 100
No: Score 5 and go to 100

**100** Does your drinking cause family rows?
Yes: Score A1, C1 and D1 and go to 101
No: Score 5 and go to 101

**101** Do you have tremors or shakes caused by drinking?
Yes: Score A1, C1 and D1 and go to 102
No: Score 5 and go to 102

**102** Does your drinking affect your memory or ability to concentrate?
Yes: Score A1, C1 and D1 and go to 103
No: Score 5 and go to 103

**103** Have you ever been arrested for drunken driving or behaviour?
Yes: Score A1, C1 and D1 and go to 104
No: Score 5 and go to 104

**104** Do you ever lie awake at night worrying?
Yes: Score S1, D1 and H1 and go to 105
No: Score 2 and go to 105

**105** Do you find it difficult to relax?
Yes: Score S1, D1 and H1 and go to 106
No: Score 2 and go to 106

**106** Do you suffer a lot from boredom?
Yes: Score S1, D1 and H1 and go to 107
No: Score 2 and go to 107

**107** Do you have too much responsibility?
Yes: Score S1, D1 and H1 and go to 108
No: Score 2 and go to 108

**108** Do you wish you had less responsibility?
Yes: Score S1, D1 and H1 and go to 109
No: Score 2 and go to 109

**109** Do you ever think that you could do more with your life?
Yes: Score S1, D1 and H1 and go to 110
No: Score 2 and go to 110

**110** Do you ever feel panicky?
Yes: Score S1, D1 and H1 and go to 111
No: Score 2 and go to 111

**111** Do you find yourself easily irritated?
Yes: Score S1, D1 and H1 and go to 112
No: Score 2 and go to 112

**112** Do you ever feel like running away from it all?
Yes: Score S1, D1 and H1 and go to 113
No: Score 2 and go to 113

**113** Are you easily annoyed by noises?
Yes: Score S1, D1 and H1 and go to 114
No: Score 2 and go to 114

**114** Do you suffer from tension headaches?
Yes: Score S1, D1 and H1 and go to 115
No: Score 2 and go to 115

**115** Do you regularly have to travel more than you like?
Yes: Score S1, D1 and H1 and go to 116
No: Score 2 and go to 116

**116** Do you regularly need to use tranquillisers?
Yes: Score S1, D1 and H1 and go to 117
No: Score 2 and go to 117

**117** Do you ever get sick or suffer from diarrhoea when you are nervous?
Yes: Score S1, D1 and H1 and go to 118
No: Score 2 and go to 118

**118** Would you describe yourself as highly strung?
Yes: Score S1, D1 and H1 and go to 119
No: Score 2 and go to 119

**119** Do you worry a lot about what other people think of you?
Yes: Score S1, D1 and H1 and go to 120
No: Score 2 and go to 120

**120** Do you worry a lot about your health?
Yes; Score S1, D1 and H1
No: Score 2

# The 20 minute health check

| | your personal score |
|---|---|
| **Health check TOTAL** | |
| **Heart disease (H)** | |
| **Respiratory disease (R)** | |
| **Digestive problems (D)** | |
| **Cancer (C)** | |
| **Muscle and joint problems (J)** | |
| **Stress susceptibility (S)** | |
| **Alcohol consumption (A)** | |

| Very unacceptable | unacceptable range | acceptable range | excellent score |
|---|---|---|---|
| 120–250 | 251–349 | 350–449 | 450+ |
| 31+ | 7–30 | 1–6 | 0 |
| 21+ | 7–20 | 1–6 | 0 |
| 21+ | 6–20 | 1–5 | 0 |
| 19+ | 6–18 | 1–5 | 0 |
| 29+ | 11–28 | 1–10 | 0 |
| 10+ | 4–9 | 1–3 | 0 |
| 4+ | 2–3 | 1 | 0 |

If any of your scores lie within the 'unacceptable' ranges, then you should turn to the appropriate advice sections which follow.

# HEALTH CHECK-SPECIFIC ADVICE

## Heart disease

Every year heart disease kills thousands of young people in their thirties and forties. The incidence of heart attacks, high blood pressure, strokes and other serious circulatory problems is also significantly higher for executives and company directors than it is for other employees.

If your assessment shows that your risk of developing heart disease or a circulatory problem is higher than it should be, then follow the advice below.

1 Limit your consumption of animal fats. There is overwhelming and indisputable evidence available to show that a high fat consumption can lead to heart disease and circulatory problems. Try to avoid fatty meat (and cut fat off meat on your plate), drink skimmed milk rather than full cream milk, avoid cream, limit your consumption of eggs to no more than three a week, and use low fat spreads instead of

butter. Use low fat alternatives for other foods whenever possible (e.g. cheese, sausages etc).

2 Keep your weight down to an acceptable level. If you need to diet then study the advice given on p. 68 .

3 You must exercise regularly but carefully. Remember that gentle exercise taken every day will do you far more good than strenuous exercise taken once or twice a week. A brisk, half hour walk every day will do far more for your health than a couple of hectic games of squash a week. See p. 75 for more details.

4 If you smoke then you should cut down your consumption of cigarettes – or better still, stop altogether. See p. 34 for advice on how to stop smoking.

5 Cut down your intake of salt. There is now evidence to show that individuals who have high blood pressure (or who are likely to develop high blood pressure) will benefit by controlling the amount of salt they consume.

## Respiratory disease

Asthma, bronchitis and other respiratory problems are a common cause of lost working time. More seriously, respiratory disorders of this type cause many deaths each year.

If your respiratory disease score was 'unacceptable' then you should take care *now* to improve your health and reduce your chances of suffering from a respiratory problem.

1 If you smoke, then you should stop. Tobacco smoke will damage your lungs and greatly increase your chances of suffering from respiratory infections. Study the advice given on p. 34 .

2 If you are overweight then you should start to diet immediately. If you carry extra, unnecessary weight then your lungs will constantly be under extra pressure. Study the advice given on p. 68 .

3 You should follow a simple, safe exercise programme in order to increase your general level of fitness. Read the advice given on p. 75 .

---

## Digestive problems

---

Indigestion is so common in our society that if five people sit down to dinner, one of them will get indigestion afterwards. And it doesn't always stop at indigestion, of course. Peptic ulceration is a common – and serious – problem which affects executives and company directors far more than other groups.

If your score lies within the unacceptable range then you need to take more care of your stomach.

Read the following advice.

1 Learn to eat slowly. People often eat far too quickly when they are under pressure. Put down your knife and fork between mouthfuls.

2 Don't try eating while you are doing something else. Only by concentrating on your eating will you be able to notice and interpret any danger or warning signs. You'll also be able to tell when you've eaten enough to satisfy your hunger – this means that you won't overload your stomach and it'll help ensure that you don't gain weight.

3 Put small amounts of food into your mouth. If you eat large mouthfuls then you'll end up failing to chew your food properly. Chewing is an essential part of the digestive process, and the saliva in your mouth contains enzymes which help prepare your food for the secretions produced by your stomach.

4 Try to taste – and enjoy – each mouthful of food. That way you're far less likely to eat too much, too quickly.

5 If you smoke then try to stop or cut down. Tobacco smoke irritates the stomach lining (see p. 34 for advice).

6 Try to keep your consumption of alcohol to a minimum. And try to avoid drinking on an empty stomach. Alcohol, like tobacco, can damage your stomach.

7 When you've finished a meal, have a short rest. Give your stomach time to digest your food before you start chasing round again.

8 Remember that regular meals are better for you than irregular meals. By eating regularly you'll be helping to mop up some of the acid in

your stomach. If you eat irregularly, the acid in your stomach will have nothing to act on – except your stomach lining.

9 Try to find out what sorts of food upset your stomach – and avoid them. Simple advice which is often ignored! It's impossible to offer a comprehensive list, but if you have an easily irritated stomach then it's likely that any of the foods on this list may exacerbate your symptoms: all fried foods; strong tea or coffee; fizzy drinks; fatty foods; spicy foods; pickles; curry; pepper; mustard; broad beans, brussels sprouts; radishes; cucumber; unripe fruit; very hot or very cold food; coarse bread; nuts; dried fruit; any tough meat that can't easily be chewed.

10. Try to minimize your exposure to stress (see p. 37).

## Cancer

Cancer is one of the two major killers of the 20th century (the other major killer is heart disease). It has replaced infectious diseases such as smallpox, typhoid and cholera as the scourge of the developed world. The very word is often enough to strike terror into most people's hearts. But cancer is not the unstoppable killer we imagine it to be. Cancer can often be prevented and it can frequently be cured.

If your cancer risk score was unacceptable then read the advice which follows. It may help save your life.

1 The commonest known cause of cancer is tobacco. If you smoke then you should either try to stop or to cut down. Remember that even cutting down will help improve your chances of avoiding cancer. See p. 34 for advice on how to cut down the amount you smoke.

2 It is now known that stress makes the development of cancer more likely. Read the advice on p. 37.

3 There is evidence to show that if you are a heavy drinker then your chances of developing cancer are increased. If you suspect that you might drink too much then read the advice notes on p. 53.

4 Be aware of the early warning signs which *can* indicate a possible cancer developing. These are:

   (a) unexplained bleeding from anywhere

   (b) any persistent change in your body (e.g. loss of weight)

   (c) a change (e.g. bleeding, colour, size) in any existing wart or skin blemish

   (d) unexplained pain which persists or recurs.

## CANCER – FOR SMOKERS ONLY

If you're a smoker you are probably already fed up with hearing of the dangers of tobacco. You probably already know that a 30-year-old who smokes just ten cigarettes a day is carving five years off his life expectancy.

But I wonder if you know just how many different diseases – in addition to cancer – are caused by cigarettes?

Here are just a few of the diseases caused or made worse by smoking: asthma, bronchitis, catarrh, sinusitis, gum and tooth disorders, indigestion, gastritis, stomach ulcers, angina, heart attacks, strokes and high blood pressure.

Even if you feel that you aren't ever going to be able to give up smoking completely you can reduce the risks by changing your smoking habits.

TRY cutting down. Twenty cigarettes a day will do less harm than forty cigarettes a day.

TRY smoking tipped cigarettes or smoking cigarettes through a holder or filter. The filter will take out some of the harmful substances.

TRY switching to low tar cigarettes – they do your health less harm.

If you want to give up smoking read the list of questions opposite – and then position them in order of their importance to you. So, if you do most of your smoking in bed, put that right at the top of the list. If you never smoke in bed put that question right at the bottom of the list.

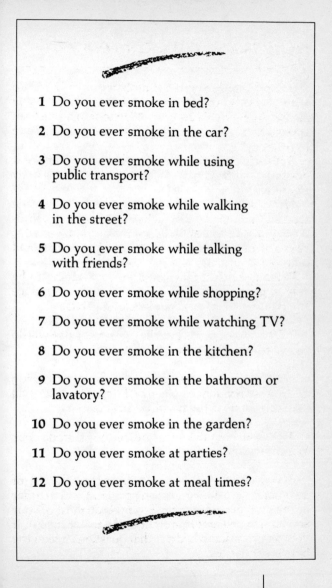

1 Do you ever smoke in bed?

2 Do you ever smoke in the car?

3 Do you ever smoke while using public transport?

4 Do you ever smoke while walking in the street?

5 Do you ever smoke while talking with friends?

6 Do you ever smoke while shopping?

7 Do you ever smoke while watching TV?

8 Do you ever smoke in the kitchen?

9 Do you ever smoke in the bathroom or lavatory?

10 Do you ever smoke in the garden?

11 Do you ever smoke at parties?

12 Do you ever smoke at meal times?

If there are any situations where you do smoke that aren't on this list then add them.

To give up smoking you must now stop smoking in each situation in turn – working your way up from the bottom of your list to the top.

So, if you smoke fewest cigarettes in the kitchen you should begin your no smoking campaign by giving up cigarettes in the kitchen. You can carry on smoking everywhere else.

When you can honestly say that you never smoke in the kitchen you can cross that question off your list and move on up your list to the next question.

You must not move upwards until you have completely given up smoking in the situation that is currently at the bottom of your list.

The advantage of this simple but effective system is that you will be able to give up smoking at a convenient and acceptable rate. And even if you can't give up smoking completely you will be able to reduce your consumption of cigarettes considerably.

Finally, remember that if you usually smoke to help you deal with stress then you must find other ways to combat stress.

# *Muscle and joint problems*

The commonest joint problem is arthritis.

Few diseases affect as many people as arthritis; few cause as much pain, discomfort and disablement. If your 'Joint' score was unacceptable then the chances are that if you don't already have arthritis, then unless you change your lifestyle, you will develop arthritis in the future.

But do not despair. The whole point of the health

check is to show you what risks you are exposed to so that you can change your lifestyle and reduce your risks.

Here are the major changes you can make.

1 Control your weight. If you are overweight then your joints will be under extra, unnecessary strain. Every extra pound of fat that you carry means that the joints of your back, hips and knees in particular, are put under unnecessary pressure. Read the advice on p. 68.

2 Learn to exercise safely and carefully. Never push yourself to the point of pain, for example. Pain is the body's way of saying 'stop'. If you insist on pushing yourself through the 'pain barrier' or if you try to 'go for the burn' in the gym, then you will damage your body – and end up with inflamed, sore joints. And take care to buy and use good equipment. Well designed shoes will help protect your feet, ankles, knees and hips. Don't run on hard roads (the shock waves can easily damage your joints). Don't run on cambered surfaces (your 'lower' leg will be under exceptional strain). Read the advice on p. 75.

## *Stress susceptibility*

Stress is the greatest environmental hazard of our time. Stress – whether produced by fear, anxiety, worry, apprehension, anger or even joy – can cause quite genuine physical responses and very real mental and physical disorders.

At a conservative estimate at least 75% of all the

problems seen by doctors are illnesses which are either completely or partly caused by stress. Staying alive today is like staying alive in the middle of a war – with stress the ever present enemy. The list of physical and mental problems caused by stress is seemingly endless – stomach ulcers, asthma, heart disease, high blood pressure, eczema – the list goes on and on.

Traditionally we often associate stress induced disease with executives and company directors. But stress doesn't just affect these groups – stress affects everyone.

If your score in the health check showed that you are susceptible to stress then you need to learn how to 'stressproof' your body.

In order to reduce the damage done to you by stress you need to be able to recognize the causes of stress and improve your own resistance.

# 1. IDENTIFY THE CAUSES OF STRESS IN YOUR LIFE

Here is my list in descending order of the ten most stressful events you are likely to have to face.

---

- ○ Death of a loved one
- ○ Divorce or separation from someone you love
- ○ Serious personal injury or illness
- ○ Moving house
- ○ Going to prison
- ○ Getting married
- ○ Being made redundant or retiring
- ○ Being pregnant or having a new baby in the house
- ○ Money worries – e.g. being in debt
- ○ Starting a new job

---

If you have experienced any of the events on this list during the last twelve months then you will have been exposed to tremendous stress.

Now make a list of all the things that YOU think could be causing stress in YOUR life. Write them all down on a piece of paper – everything that worries you, upsets you, causes you anxiety or, in your opinion, adds to the amount of stress in your life.

Next, look through your list. Just making the list –

and looking at it – will be therapeutic. And you'll be amazed to see how many of the things that are causing you stress can be solved. Some of your simpler worries can probably be solved with a phone call or a letter!

## 2. THE EARLY WARNING SIGNS OF STRESS

How do you know if you are suffering from stress? How can you tell if the pressures you are under are damaging your health?

Easy. Just look for the early warning signs which show that you have reached your stress limits.

Here are some of the commonest physical early warning signs:

○ Headaches

○ Chest Pains

○ Insomnia

○ Palpitations

○ Tiredness

○ Diarrhoea

○ Wheezing

○ Indigestion

And here are some of the mental signs which commonly occur when the pressure is too great:

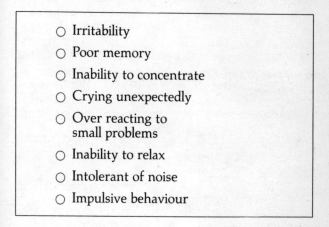

- ○ Irritability
- ○ Poor memory
- ○ Inability to concentrate
- ○ Crying unexpectedly
- ○ Over reacting to small problems
- ○ Inability to relax
- ○ Intolerant of noise
- ○ Impulsive behaviour

## 3. LEARN HOW TO RELAX YOUR BODY

When you're anxious and under stress your muscles get tense and tight. Your body responds physically to all potential threats – that's an evolutionary left-over from the days when our threats came from wild animals, not inflation, unemployment and unpaid gas bills!

Many of the physical problems associated with stress – headaches and backache for example – are caused directly by this tensing of the muscles.

You can easily reduce the damage done – and improve your resistance under pressure – by learning how to relax your body.

Many people are put off by the word 'relaxation'. Frightened, they assume it means adopting strange postures or chanting peculiar phrases over and over again! Others think that they can relax by slumping down in front of the TV set with a can of beer and the remote control button. Both are wrong. The truth is somewhere in between these two extremes.

If you can learn to swim or ride a bicycle then you can learn how to relax. Relaxation is a trick. And once you've learned to do it then the trick will stay with you for the rest of your life.

When you are learning to relax you'll need to choose a quiet, private place where you won't be disturbed – your bedroom perhaps.

Once you've mastered the art of physical relaxation you'll be able to do it anywhere!

This is what you do:

1 Lie down and make yourself as comfortable as you can. Loosen your clothes.

2 Clench your left hand as tightly as you can. Make a fist so that your knuckles go white. Now, let your fist unfold and you'll feel the muscles relax. When your hand was clenched the muscles were tensed. Unfolded the same muscles are relaxed. This is what you must do with all the muscles of your body.

3 Deliberately tense – and then relax – the muscles of your left arm. Once your left arm is relaxed let it lie loosely by your side – and ignore it.

4 Relax your right hand and arm.

5 Relax your left foot and then your left leg.

6 Relax your right foot and right leg.

7 Tense your buttock muscles. Then relax them.

8 Tense and relax your tummy muscles and then your chest muscles.

9 Tense and relax your back, shoulder and neck muscles.

10 Tense and relax all the muscles of your face. While you do all this take big, slow, deep, regular breaths. Practise this technique for 15 minutes every day.

---

## 4. LEARN HOW TO RELAX YOUR MIND

---

Under normal circumstances an almost unending stream of facts and feelings will pour into your mind. Your eyes and your ears will join with your other senses in gathering an enormous variety of bits and pieces of information.

Each one of those pieces of information will produce assessments, interpretations and conclusions.

If you can cut down the amount of information that your mind is receiving then you will cut down the number of mental responses that take place.

You will become rested and relaxed and your body and your mind will benefit in a number of ways. You will suffer far less from existing stresses and your resistance to new stresses will rise.

The most lasting and effective way to relax your mind is to learn how to daydream.

Most of us daydream when we are small. But our teachers often teach us that it is a wasteful habit. In fact, it isn't! Daydreaming – done properly – will help you relax and stay calm when the world is crumbling around you.

To daydream effectively you have to allow your imagination to dominate your thinking. Once you've learned to do it you'll be able to use the technique wherever you are and whatever you are doing.

To begin with you have to practise.

Start by finding somewhere comfortable to lie down. Get yourself as comfortable as you can. Take big deep breaths.

Now, try to conjure up some particularly restful and relaxing scene from your past.

Imagine, for example, that you are lying on a beach. Imagine that you can feel the sun on your body and the warm sand on your back. Imagine that you can hear the waves breaking on the shore and the seagulls calling high overhead.

The more realistic you can make your daydream the more relaxed you will feel.

You can, of course, use any scene you like when you are daydreaming. You can build up a library of your own private daydreams, some based on personal memories, some on books, films or TV shows.

# 5. LET YOUR EMOTIONS SHOW

Crying is a healthy response to some types of stress. It is a natural, human way of responding to sadness. When we are very young and unhappy we cry to make it clear to those who are close to us that we need sympathy and attention.

Scientists have even managed to show that when we cry through sadness our bodies are getting rid of harmful chemicals that would, if allowed to accumulate, make us feel depressed.

Crying is a useful and constructive way of dealing with personal stresses.

However, because crying is such an obvious sign of distress, many people regard it as a sign of weakness and emotional instability. Boys are taught that it is unforgivable for them to cry and that they should bottle up their feelings rather than let themselves be seen with tears on their cheeks.

Suppressing tears can, however, produce all sorts of problems. The stresses and strains will simply accumulate inside and will eventually produce genuine physical disorders.

So, my advice is that whether you are young or old, male or female, don't be afraid to let the tears flow if you can feel them coming. It is much safer, healthier and more natural to let the stress out of your body than to store it inside.

Similarly, you should also try to get rid of any anger or frustration that you feel.

Whatever causes it anger is often physically and mentally damaging. Stored, unexpressed anger will produce high blood pressure and all the other symptoms of stress induced disease.

Heart attacks, strokes and cancer are all known to be more common among people who always try to keep their anger inside their bodies.

Of course, I'm not suggesting that you should try hitting people who've annoyed you. That will merely create more problems!

But here are some tips to help you deal with anger more effectively:

1 Learn to recognize when you're heading towards a confrontation. Never be too proud to back down or apologize if you're wrong. (Sometimes, even if you're right, backing down may be the only sensible solution!).

2 Get rid of your aggression when you can. Hit a squash or tennis ball. Dig the garden. Beat a carpet. Chop up some wood. Or take a pile of old plates into the garage and smash them.

## 6. RELAX AT NIGHT – SLEEP NATURALLY

Millions of people need sleeping tablets and tranquillisers to help them get through life. But these can cause more problems than they solve. Amazingly, experts now believe that many of the drugs most commonly prescribed as sleeping pills can *cause* insomnia, *cause* anxiety, and *cause* depression! The experts certainly agree that pills of this type are never suitable for long term use.

So, here are some tips on how best you can learn to sleep naturally.

1 If you take sleeping pills don't stop them suddenly. These pills can be very addictive – they need to be stopped slowly, over a period of time. Talk to your doctor and ask for his help. If he can't or won't help you then change doctors.

2 Make sure that your bed is comfortable and that your bedroom is neither too hot nor too cold.

3 If you find yourself lying awake thinking of the day's problems, take a walk, soak in a hot bath for fifteen minutes, then go to bed with a good, relaxing book.

4 Don't worry if you seem to need less sleep than other people – or you need less sleep than you used to need. We all need different amounts of sleep and we most of us need less sleep as we get older.

5 If you still feel alert and full of life when you go to bed tire yourself out with exercise.

6 If you lie awake at night thinking about the day's problems try writing down your worries – keep a notebook by the side of your bed so that you can jot down new problems as they pop into your head.

7 If you're kept awake by other symptoms – e.g. pain or breathlessness – talk to your doctor and ask for his help. It is much better to treat the specific symptom that is keeping you awake than merely to rely on sleeping tablets.

8 If you are kept awake by noise buy some ear plugs from the chemists – they work marvellously!

9 Avoid tea or coffee last thing at night. Both can keep you awake.

10 If you are currently trying to lose weight then don't worry if you don't need to sleep as much – it's natural for slimmers to sleep less.

# 7. MISCELLANEOUS TIPS FOR STRESS CONTROL

Finally, there are some extra pieces of advice to help you deal with stress more effectively:

1 Get rid of your worries by writing them down. Buy yourself an armful of notebooks and pencils. Then write down all the problems that fill your mind. Make lists of the things you have to do. This will help you in several ways. First, once your anxieties are on paper you will be able to stop worrying about them so much. Second, when they are written down many problems seem far less significant. Tick off each problem as you have solved it and you'll be surprised and delighted to find that some problems will have sorted themselves out before you've got round to ticking them off. When you've got a really tricky problem to solve write down all the possible solutions you can think of and add to the list as new solutions occur to you. Eventually, you'll find that one particular solution will stand out as the only practicable answer.

2 Put purpose into your life. Having a purpose will enable you to live through the worst of life's crises. Begin by making a list of all the goals and ambitions you had when you were a teenager. Try to think back and remember what hopes and aspirations fired your imagination at that age. Then take a look through your list to see just how many of those

dreams still excite you. Many of your old dreams are probably still within reach.

3 Sort out your priorities. If you fail to differentiate between the big problems and the little ones you will suffer in several ways. First, small worries will take your mind off important problems – with devastating long term consequences. Second, the sheer number of problems you're exposed to will damage your health. Try to decide what is really important to you. Try to see things in perspective. Don't be fooled into wasting time on things that are really not important to you.

4 Kiss and cuddle the people you love. Insurance companies in America have shown that if a wife kisses her husband before he goes off to work then he will, on average, live five years longer than if he doesn't get a good morning kiss. Try not to hide your feelings for those whom you love.

5 Put more laughter into your life. Laughter is a positive, natural phenomenon which can really help you to stay healthy. Laughter helps by improving respiration, lowering blood pressure and 'tuning up' the heart. To put more laughter into your life make sure that you spend more time with cheerful, happy people and keep a library of your favourite funny books or films so that you can cheer yourself up when you're feeling miserable.

6 Build up your self confidence. A lack of self confidence can mean that you push yourself too hard – and become very susceptible to outside

pressures. Try imagining that you are writing an advertisement for yourself. Make a list of all your best points. Pick out of the following list the adjectives that can be applied to you:

careful, moral, kind, generous, ambitious, hard working, creative, fair, thoughtful, attentive, honest, conscientious, unselfish, tolerant, friendly, considerate, soft-hearted, good-humoured, charitable, witty, wise, clever.

Next time you're feeling a failure look at the list you made and you'll see that you're not such a disaster after all.

7 Learn to assert yourself. People who allow themselves to be pushed around suffer far more from stress than more assertive individuals. You don't have to be aggressive, rude or unpleasant. Simply try to be aware of your own needs and wishes – and be more prepared to stand your ground. Learn to stand up for yourself. Learn to say 'no' when you really don't want to do something. You'll find that other people will treat you with more respect and consideration. You'll also suffer far less from stress.

8 Remember that boredom can cause stress. If you feel that your life is too dull then take up a pastime or hobby which you find rewarding. Do something that you can take a pride in. Start evening classes at a local college. And be prepared to take risks occasionally – even if it means a few failures.

9 Buy yourself a rocking chair. When I was small I used to go and visit an old aunt who had a massive, old-fashioned rocking chair. I noticed

that when she was upset she would rock herself slightly faster than usual. It was almost as though she was using the rocking chair to soothe her troubled nerves. It now seems that that was exactly what she was doing. The rhythmic motion helps by counteracting urgent 'help' messages being sent out by the brain. The rocking chair is a wooden tranquilliser that can help relax the body and brain and drain away accumulated tensions.

10 Don't be afraid to complain. If the Government plans to build a nuclear plant behind your home start a petition. Write to your local newspaper. Let your feelings be known. Complaining may not always get you the results you want – but it will help minimize the feelings of frustration that can cause so much damage.

11 Learn how to deal with panic attacks. The ordinary symptoms associated with anxiety – butterflies in the stomach, palpitations, headache, shaking hands, dry mouth – are all bad enough. But occasionally these symptoms build up and produce a 'panic attack'. If you get such an attack take a huge breath, hold it just as long as you can, let it out slowly and then take another really big, deep breath to replace it. Continue these deep breathing exercises for as long as is necessary.

12 Take a break occasionally. When you are feeling shattered and the stress in your life is intolerable take a break – grab a few days and go somewhere to unwind. If you've got small children, try to park them with friends or relatives for a few days. They won't suffer for a

day or two. Indeed, they'll benefit if you come back relaxed and less irritable. If you have difficulty in finding someone to look after the children try to fix up a reciprocal arrangement with another couple – perhaps a pair with children a similar age to your own. That way they can look after your children while you have a break – and then you can look after theirs in return. And when you go away do go somewhere peaceful. Don't try to see 14 countries in 3 days or else you'll come back home even more stressed!

## Alcohol consumption

If your score fell short of acceptable then your drinking habits could soon lead to serious problems.

Alcoholism is a major problem today – among women as well as men.

Many people still believe that the only organ likely to be damaged by drinking is the liver – that isn't true. People who drink heavily risk developing cancer, stomach ulcers and muscle wastage too. Women who drink too much and get pregnant run a real risk of having backward or low birthweight babies. They are more at risk of liver disease than men because the female body is physiologically more vulnerable to alcohol than the male body.

Apart from the physical effects, however, it is the effects it has on the brain that make alcohol particularly dangerous.

Alcohol is detectable in the brain within half a minute of a glass being emptied. Basically, alcohol is a depressant. It depresses normal inhibitions and it depresses reflexes. The individual who has had a few drinks will think that he or she is able to talk coherently or drive a motor car well but, in fact, his or her ability to do either of those things will be badly affected.

Here are some staggering facts about the damage done by alcohol:

- Alcohol causes between a third and a half of all road deaths.

- A third of all accidents at work are caused by alcohol.

- One fifth of all male admissions to general medical wards are related to the use of alcohol.

- Up to three quarters of police time is spent on alcohol related crimes.

- Between a third and a half of all the individuals admitted to psychiatric hospitals need in-patient help because they drink too much.

- If you are an alcoholic you are around four times as likely to die in any given year than a non-drinker of the same age, sex and economic status. You are more likely to be involved in serious accidents, to suffer from liver trouble and to develop cancer. An alcoholic is more likely to be involved in a violent crime than a social drinker or non-drinker. And an alcoholic runs the risk of suffering from serious and permanent brain damage.

Here is the health check plan for controlling your drinking:

1 Read through questions 94 to 103 carefully. See where you accumulated most of your 'A' points. You should be able to learn something about the consequences of your personal drinking habits from these questions.

2 You need help, support and guidance now. Get in touch with the local branch of Alcoholics Anonymous (the telephone number will be in the 'phone book) and ask for their help.

3 Do not make the mistake of saying that you can 'kick it later'. Alcohol is a drug – a dangerously addictive drug.

4 Learn how to deal with stress and pressure more effectively – particularly if you are accustomed to drinking when you are under pressure. Read the notes on p. 37.

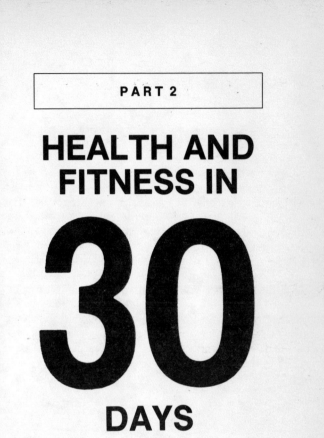

## PART 2

# HEALTH AND FITNESS IN

# 30

# DAYS

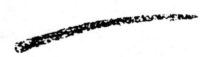

# *INTRODUCTION*

Don't be too alarmed if your health check score fell into one of the 'unacceptable' ranges – or if you failed to obtain 'excellent' scores in all categories. The whole point of completing the check is to find out how good or bad your current lifestyle is – and to spot potential problems now!

If you want to improve your health and fitness then read the advice on the following pages. If you follow my advice you'll obtain a permanent improvement! You'll look good and feel better!

In just 30 days you'll notice a real change in your health – a change that you can actually *measure!*

But, more important, you'll have acquired good habits that can change your life for ever.

# PRESCRIPTION NUMBER 1

## Improve your eating habits

The wrong foods can kill you just as surely as a bullet.

Few things have as important an effect on your health as the food you choose to eat. Your body is, after all, *made* from the food you eat.

Many so-called experts have made sensible eating sound unnecessarily complicated – often because they're trying to sell you special products in which they have a vested interest.

In fact the truth is very simple.

## RULE NO 1: CUT DOWN YOUR FAT CONSUMPTION

Most of us eat far too much fatty food – and it often makes us ill. If you eat large amounts of animal fat then you run a higher than average risk of having a heart attack.

The first link between fat intake and heart disease was noticed over thirty years ago. Since then dozens of highly respected authorities have reported that when people eat less fat they have fewer heart attacks. Animal fats, say the experts, are a major threat to your health.

To reduce your risk of having a heart attack or a stroke (and remember that more people die of heart disease than any other disease – including *all* the cancers put together) follow these straightforward rules to help keep your fat intake to a minimum:

1 Grill rather than fry your food. Adding extra fat to foods such as bacon that already have a high fat content is hazardous to your health.

2 Eat less fatty meat. When shopping try to buy lean cuts of meat. If you buy meat with fat attached then cut it off either before cooking or before eating.

3 Try not to eat more than two or three eggs a week.

4 Avoid top of the cream milk and full cream milk. You're much safer with skimmed milk.

5 Don't use butter or hard margarine. Instead use low fat spreads or spreads containing polyunsaturates.

6 Cook with corn oil or sunflower oil – this way you can make chips that won't damage your health.

Finally, remember that the big companies and farmers who want to sell you fatty foods will continue to buy advertising space designed to persuade you to buy *more* butter, milk and cream!

Don't let them weaken your resolve. They're just after your money. If you want to stay healthy then follow my advice!

---

## RULE NO. 2: INCREASE THE AMOUNT OF FIBRE YOU EAT

---

Fibre is an essential part of your diet. If you don't have enough fibre you'll be more likely to suffer from gallstones, diabetes, appendicitis, varicose veins and a huge range of bowel disorders.

But for years now food manufacturers have been taking all the roughage out of our food. Originally this was done because roughage didn't contain any nutrients – it simply goes through the intestines unchanged. Then slowly scientists realized that roughage is essential!

Over several million years our digestive systems have been developed in such a way that the roughage has an important part to play. It is the roughage that helps to keep food moving through your intestines.

Without the roughage – the fibre – we develop an enormous list of dangerous and uncomfortable diseases. So, how do you increase the amount of fibre you eat? Simple!

Eat more: fresh fruit, fresh vegetables (particularly peas and beans), brown rice, nuts, digestive biscuits and potatoes in their skins. Eat brown or wholemeal bread and use wholemeal flour when baking.

And remember that baked beans contain more fibre than any other modern convenience foods! Baked beans on wholemeal bread really are good for you.

Finally, there is one more advantage to be gained by eating more fibre – it will help you slim!

Fibre helps you stay slim because although it makes you feel full quicker it contains little that can be absorbed and stored as fat.

---

## RULE NO. 3: CUT OUT SUGAR

---

Dental decay is one of the commonest of all diseases. Dentists remove several tons of teeth every year – nearly a third of all British adults have lost all their teeth. Sugar is the main cause of all this tooth rot.

Sugar will also make you fat and endanger your health in other ways.

And yet despite the fact that we often consider sugar to be an 'essential' food (it is usually one of the first foodstuffs parachuted in when outlying villages are cut off by floods or snow) we can live quite well without sugar.

If you have already acquired a taste for sweet things try using artificial sweeteners – in cooking and in drinks – instead of sugar.

Despite some scares a few years ago the sweeteners on the market now are probably less likely to kill you than sugar.

And remember that children aren't usually born with a 'sweet tooth' – it's a habit they acquire. When children want a snack give them fruit or fresh vegetables to chew rather than bags of sticky sweets. And when they grow up encourage them to drink their tea or coffee without added sugar.

# RULE NO. 4: KEEP UP YOUR VITAMINS

More nonsense is talked about vitamins than about anything else we eat. According to the claims I've seen vitamin supplements are said to cure diseases ranging from bad eyesight to arthritis. Some of the claims made for vitamins are simply untrue and others are based on flimsy, disputable or rocky evidence.

The plain truth is that if you eat a good, sensible, balanced diet you will automatically get the vitamins and minerals your body needs.

And extra vitamin supplements won't make you any healthier – any more than pumping an extra million volts into your TV set will give you a better picture. Indeed, too many vitamin tablets can *harm* your health! So, get your vitamins naturally – from the food you eat.

Vitamin A is found in milk, eggs, butter, margarine, cheese, liver, fish oils and carrots.

Vitamin B (which actually consists of several different substances) is found in many different foods. You'll get all you need if you eat a good and varied diet which includes some cereals.

Vitamin C is available in fruits and vegetables. Remember not to overcook vegetables.

Vitamin D is present in cheese, butter, margarine and liver. There is also enough sunshine in most parts of the world to provide the majority of us with all the vitamin D we need.

Vitamin E has been described as the vitamin in search of a disease! Vitamin E is so common that anyone who eats a diet low in vitamin E will die of something else long before the vitamin E deficiency can cause any symptoms.

So much for vitamins – what about minerals? Again the truth is that if you eat a good, well-balanced diet then you will get the minerals your body needs.

Remember – if you really think your body needs vitamin or mineral supplements then you should see your doctor. First, to find out why your body is short of these essentials and secondly, to make sure that the shortage is remedied accurately and scientifically.

## RULE NO. 5: TAKE CARE WITH SALT

It has been known for many years that people with a family history of high blood pressure are more likely to develop problems if they eat too much salt. And since 1941 it has been known that a low salt diet can help high blood pressure sufferers.

A low salt diet can also help people who retain water – for example, women who swell up just before a period.

If you think that you would benefit by reducing the amount of salt in your diet then avoid the following foods (or, at least, keep your consumption of them down to a minimum):

○ processed foods in general

○ canned foods

○ junk foods (such as takeaway hamburgers)

○ crisps

○ salted peanuts

○ cheese crackers

○ chips

○ lobsters

○ oysters

○ salted butter and cheese

○ sausages

○ bacon

○ milk products

You should also avoid adding salt when cooking food. And salt should be banished from your table.

If you find saltless food unappetizing there are a number of other flavourings that you can try. These include; lemon juice, parsley, garlic, horseradish, and tarragon.

---

## AND FINALLY ...

---

1 Don't worry too much about cholesterol. You *can* cut down your consumption of cholesterol by cutting down on foods that contain cholesterol (cheese, chocolate, cream, eggs, hearts, kidneys, brains, caviare, liver, shellfish and sweetbreads) but if you keep your consumption of fat down you'll probably be doing all that's necessary since fats are converted into cholesterol in your body.

2 To reduce your consumption of food additives buy as much fresh food as you can. But don't worry about additives too much – the problems they create has been exaggerated in recent years.

3 Remember that both tea and coffee contain caffeine – a powerful stimulant. In small quantities caffeine won't do you any harm but in large quantities it can prove addictive. If, when you wake up in the morning, you *have* to drink a cup of tea or coffee before you start the day then you may be a caffeine addict. Watch out too if you drink more than half a dozen cups of either a day, if you feel uncomfortable if you go for several hours without a drink or if you frequently suffer from unexplained symptoms such as headaches or tiredness. To cut down

your intake of caffeine drink fewer cups, make weaker drinks (remember that ground coffee contains more caffeine than instant coffee and that coffee contains more caffeine than tea) or drink decaffeinated products.

4 When buying sausages and meat pies look for products that have lower than normal fat contents.

5 Remember that chicken and other poultry are lower in animal fat than other meats. And don't forget fish when you're shopping.

6 Don't assume that in order to buy healthy food you have to shop at a 'health food' shop. This just isn't true. Many so called 'health food' shops sell foods that are no better than the ordinary foods sold (usually at lower prices) in other shops and supermarkets. If you want to find good, wholesome foods at reasonable prices look around all the local shops and check out the labelling, the prices and the freshness of the products on sale. Some big supermarkets are now well aware of the demand for good quality healthy food. Look around and you may well be surprised.

7 Remember that a *little* of what you fancy will probably do you good – its unlikely to do you much harm!

# PRESCRIPTION NUMBER 2

## Keep your weight under control

In half the world the majority of illnesses which kill and disable are caused – or made worse – by a lack of food.

In the other half of the world – the half in which you and I live – the majority of illnesses are caused by or made worse by our eating too much food.

It is impossible to work out precisely how many people die because they are overweight – but there isn't a shadow of doubt that obesity is a major cause of death.

If you are overweight you are more likely to get high blood pressure, develop heart disease, have a stroke or develop diabetes. In addition obesity is likely to make your life unpleasant and uncomfortable. It makes crippling diseases such as asthma and arthritis far worse than they need be – and it commonly causes mental problems such as anxiety and depression.

The truth, however, is that by following my simple rules you can not only lose any excess, unwanted weight but you can also stay slim for ever.

In the advice which follows I haven't included a list of foods that you must not eat for the simple reason that it is not *WHAT* you eat that determines your weight so much as *HOW MUCH* you eat. Acquiring new eating habits is a far healthier and wiser way to lose weight than slavishly following an unnatural (and probably unhealthy) diet.

## *The basic facts*

Food is the fuel which helps keep your body alive. It is food that keeps your muscles moving, your brain buzzing and your heart beating.

Food is burnt up all the time and the rate at which it disappears depends on exactly what you are doing.

Push your body hard and you'll burn up more food.

Lie in bed and you'll burn up less food.

It is the relationship between the amount of food your body *needs* and the amount of food you *eat* that decides whether you put on weight, lose weight or stay the same.

If you eat less food than your body needs you'll have to burn up stored food from your fat deposits to keep going. You'll lose weight. If you eat more food than your body needs you'll have food to spare and the spare will be stored as fat – you'll gain weight. Eat exactly what your body needs and your weight will stay stable.

There are, consequently, two basic ways of losing weight.

1 You can increase the amount of work you do – and burn up food faster than you are taking it in.

2 You can reduce your intake of food below your body's requirements.

In either case your body will have to take food from your stored fat deposits to satisfy its need for energy.

The first of these two techniques – doing more exercise – sounds attractive but it doesn't work very well. To lose a pound of fat you have to do an enormous amount of exercise. Exercise will help you diet but it isn't the sole answer.

The only real solution is to eat less than your body needs. But, to many people that means going hungry. And it can be uncomfortable. It's hardly surprising that so many diets fail.

Here are the simple rules that will change your life for ever. Follow these eating guidelines and you'll get slim and stay slim.

---

## RULE 1

---

Only ever eat when you are hungry. And stop eating when you are no longer hungry. Every time you are about to put food into your mouth ask yourself these two simple questions: 'Am I really hungry? Do I need this?'

If you can learn to eat when you are hungry then this will be the last time in your life that you ever need to diet.

---

## RULE 2

---

Set yourself manageable targets. Work out how much you need to lose. Then aim to lose 8 pounds a month – just 2 pounds a week. That doesn't sound much but if you keep to the same rate of weight loss you will have lost 96 pounds in a year – that's nearly 7 stones!

By giving yourself monthly targets for weight loss you will find dieting easier. And every time you 'hit' your target your confidence will be boosted.

## RULE 3

Try to eat lots of foods – such as raw vegetables – that need a lot of chewing. Foods that take time will slow you down and make you eat less. Eating slowly really is important. Put down your knife and fork between mouthfuls to slow yourself down even more.

## RULE 4

When you feel hungry eat filling but low calorie snacks. A cup of black coffee or lemon tea, a one calorie cola drink or a bowl of clear soup will help assuage your hunger without putting calories into your body. If you need something more filling try baked beans on wholemeal bread – really filling but relatively low in calories.

## RULE 5

If you are planning a big meal have a small snack half an hour beforehand. It doesn't matter what – an apple, a raw carrot or a low calorie drink. The idea is to fill your stomach so that your appetite will be spoilt. When you start eating you won't feel quite as hungry as you might otherwise have felt. You can even 'spoil' your appetite with a glass of water.

## RULE 6

If you must have a late night snack make sure it is low in calories but filling – choose an apple or a piece of celery and a portion of low fat cheese instead of half a packet of biscuits.

## RULE 7

When you put food onto a plate spread it around to make it look as though there is a lot there – and choose small plates.

## RULE 8

Never eat other people's left overs. Don't turn yourself into a human dustbin.

## RULE 9

Try not to eat late at night (after 7 or 8 pm). Your body probably won't need the calories and they will be converted directly into fat. If you feel peckish before you go to bed have a low calorie drink.

## RULE 10 ✓

When eating out don't let politeness ruin your good eating habits. If you've had enough to eat then say so – and be prepared to leave food that you can't eat. Say 'no' to second helpings you don't really need. And don't feel guilty about saying 'no'.

## RULE 11 ✓

Get into the habit of throwing food away. When we are small we are taught that it is a sin to throw food away. We are encouraged to eat up everything in sight. But your body simply turns unwanted food into fat. The only way to beat this bad habit is to practise throwing out unwanted food. Try it now. Go into the kitchen and look through your cupboards and your fridge. Throw out all the unwanted and stale bits of food. Throw it into the dustbin or, if you've got a garden start a compost heap.

## RULE 12 ✓

Get rid of all your clothes as you lose weight. Or have them altered. Burn your boats. If you keep oversized dresses or suits in your wardrobe then you're admitting to yourself that you might put weight back on again. If you don't have anything to wear you have an added incentive to stay slim.

## RULE 13

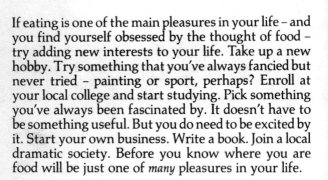

When you go out of the house don't take any spare cash for sweets, crisps, buns or other unnecessary extras. If you go into a coffee shop with just enough cash for a coffee you won't be able to buy a doughnut will you?

## RULE 14

If eating is one of the main pleasures in your life – and you find yourself obsessed by the thought of food – try adding new interests to your life. Take up a new hobby. Try something that you've always fancied but never tried – painting or sport, perhaps? Enroll at your local college and start studying. Pick something you've always been fascinated by. It doesn't have to be something useful. But you do need to be excited by it. Start your own business. Write a book. Join a local dramatic society. Before you know where you are food will be just one of *many* pleasures in your life.

# PRESCRIPTION NUMBER 3

## *Get yourself fit*

Some of the claims made for exercise have been exaggerated. Exercise won't make you sexier or brainier. And exercise alone won't help you to a slimmer, shapelier body. But exercise is essential – and if you feel fit then you'll not only be healthier but you'll feel better and brighter too.

If you take no exercise at all then your health will undoubtedly deteriorate. You will be particularly likely to suffer from problems such as heart disease and high blood pressure.

Regular, gentle exercise will help to keep your body supple and help to keep your joints mobile.

Exercise regularly and you can help minimize your chances of developing problems such as backache and muscle tension.

Exercise will not get rid of wrinkles or improve the size of your bust. Star actresses don't get their good looks and shapely figures by sweating on the gym floor every day. But exercise can firm up muscles, help hold in flab and make you look at your best.

To benefit from exercise you don't have to do anything complicated – simple, regular exercise is all you need.

## Fitness check

Check your general fitness with one of the following simple, fitness testing programmes.

1 Find a step that is about 12 inches deep and a watch that is calibrated in seconds. Then climb up and down the step 24 times a minute for a total of 3 minutes. When you've finished rest for 30 seconds and take your pulse. Your pulse rate is your score for this exercise.

2 Measure a distance of one mile on a local map. Then find out how long it takes you to cover that distance under your own steam – you can walk, jog, run, hop, skip or dance – it's up to you. Remember to make a careful note of the route you use. It is more important that you can follow the same route in future than that it is exactly one mile.

   Use a watch that is calibrated in seconds to time yourself. Your score is your time in seconds divided by 10. (So, if a mile takes you 12 minutes that is 720 seconds so your score is 72.) Measure your score to the nearest whole number.

## Note

Do *not* test your fitness if you are receiving medical treatment of any kind, if you have any symptoms or illnesses, if you are in any doubt about your general health or if a medical adviser has warned you to avoid exercise. If you are in any doubt see or telephone your doctor and ask for his advice.

Whichever testing programme you choose keep a record of your score. Then repeat the testing programme once a week. Over a period of a month or more you should be able to notice a steady but noticeable improvement in your level of fitness if you follow my advice.

# The fitness programme

## RULE 1 ✓

Once you've started an exercise programme it is important not to stop. If you are going to maintain the improvement in your fitness and general health then you must continue to exercise regularly. If you do continue with your exercise programme there is no doubt that you will benefit.

Not long ago a professor at the London School of Hygiene and Tropical Medicine published a report showing just how valuable exercise can be in helping to ward off heart trouble.

The professor and his team questioned 16,882 British civil servants aged between 40 and 64 and assessed their exercise habits. They then waited to see which civil servants had heart attacks.

They discovered that while only 11% of the civil servants who had been in the habit of taking regular exercise had heart disease no less than 26% of those who did not take exercise succumbed to heart attacks.

Exercise, they showed, improves the efficiency and effectiveness of all the muscles – including the muscles of the heart. Further the experts went on to suggest that swimming, dancing, tennis and hill climbing were among the most effective forms of exercise.

The size and power of the muscle cells improves – and the muscles develop extra blood vessels. As a result of these improvements stamina increases and there is a greater tolerance to sudden exercise. A dash for the bus or a run upstairs when the lift is out of order becomes far less of an ordeal.

There is no doubt that although too much exercise can be bad for you, exercise does improve your general health. People who are reasonably fit fall ill less frequently, are better able to cope with mental problems and with stress, get better quicker when they are ill and feel and look brighter.

## RULE 2

The best and most effective forms of exercise are often the simplest. The simplest of all forms of exercise is walking. You can start getting fit by getting off the bus a stop early, by leaving the car at home occasionally and by using the stairs instead of the lift at work. A brisk half hour walk a day will give you all the steady exercise you need.

## RULE 3

Whatever form of exercise you choose make sure that it is something you can enjoy. If exercise becomes a chore it is more likely to do you harm than good.

## RULE 4

If you are receiving medical treatment for any condition – or you have the slightest doubts about your health – see a doctor before starting any exercise programme.

---

## RULE 5 ✓

---

Ignore any so called 'experts' who say that you should try to force your way through the pain barrier. That really is dangerous nonsense. Pain is a natural defence mechanism. It is your body's way of saying STOP. If you push yourself through the pain barrier then you may well injure yourself. Remember: if it hurts – STOP.

---

## RULE 6 ✓

---

You don't have to spend lots of money – or even leave your home – to benefit from exercise. You can get all the exercise you need for the price of a pair of decent walking shoes, a swimming costume, some dancing shoes or an old bicycle.

Here is one exercise that you can try that won't cost you a penny – all you need is a flight of stairs.

Climbing stairs uses up a lot of energy and exercises all the right muscles. Scientists have shown that 50 years of stair climbing in an average house uses up the same amount of energy that would be needed to send a one ton space capsule 100 miles into the sky.

As long as you are happy about your general health – and you don't have any pains or symptoms or need to take any prescribed medicine – try this:

Go up and down one flight of stairs three or four

times in the morning. And then do the same in the afternoon. You can gradually increase this until you are going up and down ten or twelve times in each session.

If you live in a bungalow and you haven't got any stairs then look around – you'll soon find a flight at work, at the train station or in the local multi storey car park. Use the stairs instead of the lift occasionally.

Stair exercise is particularly good for two reasons:

1  Your body gets a chance to rest every time you go back downstairs again.

2  Stair climbing is excellent for your figure. The parts of your body that will benefit most are your hips, waist and bottom.

---

## RULE 7

Don't allow yourself to become too competitive unless you want to be competitive. If you are always pushing yourself to beat your previous best, to jog further or faster than you have ever jogged before or to thrash your neighbour on the squash court you'll be adding to the stress in your life. If you need more stress, that is fine. The chances are that you don't.

---

## RULE 8

Regular, gentle exercise is much better for you than violent, occasional exercise. Half an hour a day spent walking will do you much more good than a day a week spent in the gymnasium or on the squash court.

---

## RULE 9

---

If you want to make new friends and enjoy a better social life then pick your sport carefully. Golf, tennis, swimming and dancing are all excellent ways to meet new friends. You're not likely to have many sparkling conversations while sitting in a rowing machine in your bedroom.

---

## RULE 10

---

Remember that fitness is not the same as good health. Just because you can run a mile in four minutes you are not necessarily healthy. If you spend all day crouched over your exercise bicycle then at the end of a few months you will have become very good at riding your exercise bicycle. But you will not be exceptionally healthy.

---

## RULE 11

---

You can have too much exercise – and exercise can damage your health. Doctors at one British hospital recently kept a record of patients needing treatment after exercise. In one six week period 350 patients turned up injured after exercise. Some had permanently damaged their bodies. Some types of exercise – jogging and road running for example – seem particularly likely to produce injuries. But don't let the hazards put you off exercise completely – if you do no exercise at all then you'll be at real risk of killers like heart disease.

## RULE 12

Do you want to see how fit you are becoming? If so, try this.

Persuade a friend to hold on to your ankles while you lie on your back on the floor. Then clasp your hands behind your head and try to sit up, keeping your knees bent so that your thigh and lower leg form an angle of ninety degrees.

Now, touch your right knee with your left elbow.

Lie down, pull yourself up and continue with the exercise.

Alternate by touching your left knee with your right elbow.

Count the number of times that you make contact in one minute.

The average man will manage 20 to 30 of these movements in one minute.

A fit man will do more and an unfit man will do less.

The average woman will manage a similar number but the total range will be greater – a very fit woman will probably manage 50 while an overweight or unfit woman may only manage two or three.

If you want to see how your fitness is improving keep a weekly record showing many of these you manage.

# Sports – a quick guide

Here is my quick guide to the most popular forms of exercise and sport.

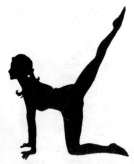

### *Aerobics*
Group activity under supervision for people who don't know how to exercise. Can be fun but potentially damaging if overdone. Sometimes taken far too seriously. Some people find it boring. Common problem is that class leader knows no more about exercise – and the potential hazards – than pupils.

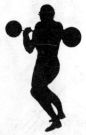

### *Body building*
You won't get sand kicked in your face and you can win prizes if you spend your time body building. But it does little or nothing for your general health.

### *Boxing and other contact sports*
The advantage is that you can get rid of all your stress by hitting somebody senseless. Disadvantage is that he might hit you first.

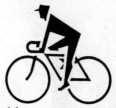

### *Cycling*
Good, simple, healthy exercise – one of my Top Four (along with dancing, swimming and walking). But take care on busy roads.

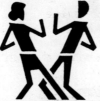

### *Dancing*
Pleasant, sociable way to get your exercise. Lots of fun.

### *Gardening*
One of the most popular ways to get regular exercise. But back injuries are common.

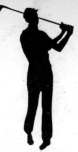

### *Golf*

As long as you don't use an electric trolley you can get a fair amount of gentle, safe exercise.

### *Jogging and running*

Overrated and overpromoted form of exercise. Not particularly good for your health – joggers often suffer joint and back troubles.

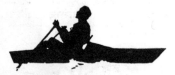

### *Rowing*

Pleasant enough if there are just two of you on the lake. But fairly deadly if you're sitting in a boat with seven others – and staring at the back of someone else's head. Even worse if you simply sit on a rowing machine.

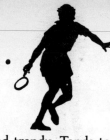

## *Squash*

Fashionable and trendy. Tends to involve bursts of wild activity rather than gentle sustained exercise. Not good for people who aren't already fit.

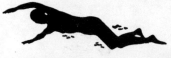

## *Swimming*

Excellent way to get good, regular exercise. Good for the elderly, disabled and overweight.

## *Tennis*

Easy way to get exercise during summer months.

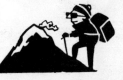

## *Walking*

Safe, enjoyable, cheap and suitable for all year round. You can do it anywhere, with anyone and at your own pace. You can get all the exercise your body needs if you exercise regularly.

# Height/weight chart (women)

### Instructions for weighing yourself

1. Weigh yourself with as few clothes as possible and no shoes.

2 Measure your height in bare or stockinged feet.

3 You are overweight if you weight falls above your ideal weight band. You are underweight if your weight falls below your ideal weight band.

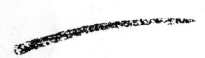

| Height (feet & inches) | Ideal Weight Band (stones and pounds) | Average Weight (stones and pounds) |
| --- | --- | --- |
| 4.10 | 7.5 – 8.5 | 7.12 |
| 4.11 | 7.7 – 8.7 | 8.0 |
| 5.0 | 7.9 – 8.9 | 8.2 |
| 5.1 | 7.11– 8.11 | 8.4 |
| 5.2 | 8.1 – 9.1 | 8.8 |
| 5.3 | 8.4 – 9.4 | 8.11 |
| 5.4 | 8.6 – 9.6 | 8.13 |
| 5.5 | 8.10– 9.10 | 9.3 |
| 5.6 | 9.0 –10.0 | 9.7 |
| 5.7 | 9.3 –10.3 | 9.10 |
| 5.8 | 9.7 –10.7 | 10.0 |
| 5.9 | 9.10–10.10 | 10.3 |
| 5.10 | 10.0 –11.0 | 10.7 |
| 5.11 | 10.3 –11.3 | 10.10 |
| 6.0 | 10.7 –11.7 | 11.0 |
| 6.1 | 10.9 –11.9 | 11.2 |
| 6.2 | 10.12–11.12 | 11.5 |
| 6.3 | 11.2 –12.2 | 11.9 |
| 6.4 | 11.5 –12.5 | 11.12 |
| 6.5 | 11.8 –12.8 | 12.1 |
| 6.6 | 12.0 –13.0 | 12.7 |

# Height/weight chart (men)

## Instructions for weighing yourself

1 Weigh yourself with as few clothes as possible and no shoes.

2 Measure your height in bare or stockinged feet.

3 You are overweight if you weight falls above your ideal weight band. You are underweight if your weight falls below your ideal weight band.

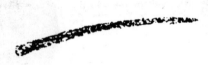

| Height (feet & inches) | Ideal Weight Band (stones and pounds) | Average Weight (stones and pounds) |
|---|---|---|
| 5.0 | 8.5 – 9.5 | 8.12 |
| 5.1 | 8.6 – 9.6 | 8.13 |
| 5.2 | 8.7 – 9.7 | 9.0 |
| 5.3 | 8.8 – 9.8 | 9.1 |
| 5.4 | 8.11– 9.11 | 9.4 |
| 5.5 | 9.2 –10.2 | 9.9 |
| 5.6 | 9.6 –10.6 | 9.13 |
| 5.7 | 9.10–10.10 | 10.3 |
| 5.8 | 10.0 –11.0 | 10.7 |
| 5.9 | 10.4 –11.4 | 10.11 |
| 5.10 | 10.8 –11.8 | 11.1 |
| 5.11 | 10.12–11.12 | 11.5 |
| 6.0 | 11.2 –12.2 | 11.9 |
| 6.1 | 11.6 –12.6 | 11.13 |
| 6.2 | 11.10–12.10 | 12.3 |
| 6.3 | 12.0 –13.0 | 12.7 |
| 6.4 | 12.4 –13.4 | 12.11 |
| 6.5 | 12.8 –13.8 | 13.1 |
| 6.6 | 13.0 –14.0 | 13.7 |

# STRESS MANAGEMENT TECHNIQUES

Managing people

for healthy profits

**Dr Vernon Coleman**

In an average lifetime the average employee loses one and a half years from work because of stress-induced illness. The result is that stress costs British industry £20 million a year – far more than is lost through strikes or industrial disputes.

'Britain,' says Dr Vernon Coleman, 'leads the world in expensive, stress-induced disease'. He points out that if a company employs just 100 people then stress will cost that company around £400 a day. In a company which employs 1,000 people stress costs £1 million a year.

Whatever else you try, and however much you spend on equipment, nothing will improve your company's efficiency and profitability more than taking care of your employees and reducing their unnecessary exposure to stress.

In *Stress Management Techniques* Dr Vernon Coleman explains exactly how, why and when stress causes problems. More importantly, he also explains exactly how you can control and minimise the amount of stress in your company.

**Mercury**  **£9.95** (Hardback)

Available from all good Bookshops.

# FIT FOR BUSINESS

A practical look

at fitness for the busy

executive

by Matthew Archer

There is ample evidence that achieving physical fitness not only improves the chances of living longer but also makes people more efficient – mentally as well as physically.

The benefits of physical exercise, sensible eating and adopting a particular lifestyle and attitude can improve the effectiveness of the business executive and provide a defence against stress-related problems.

To achieve this kind of fitness and to maintain it require no great agony. The executive who travels on business, eats working lunches and is subject to pressure need not adopt the regime of an Olympic athlete or try to live on a diet of muesli and vitamin pills. This book, written by a fitness executive, takes the fitness question apart and puts it together again in a practical form which busy executives can use.

**Mercury**   **£11.95** (Hardback)

Available from all good Bookshops.

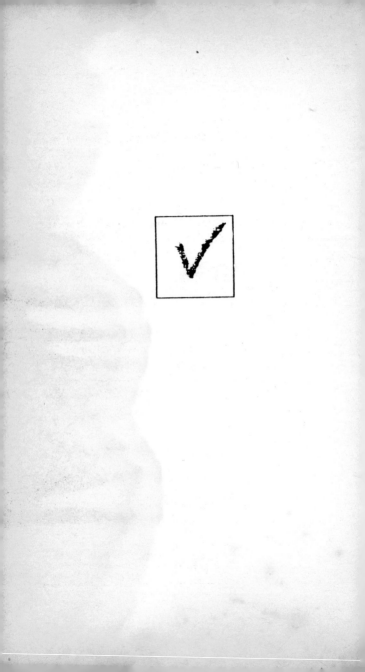

# Dr Vernon Coleman

Dr Vernon Coleman has written more than 35 books which have sold well over a million copies and regularly appear on the bestseller lists. His books are now as popular abroad as they are in the United Kingdom and have been translated into twelve languages. A qualified doctor, former family doctor and fellow of the Royal Society of Medicine, Vernon Coleman has written and presented over a dozen television and radio series based on his books and has made a great many appearances on television and radio stations in many countries. His newspaper and magazine columns make him the most widely read health writer in Britain.

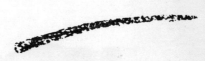